Food for Pregnancy Volume 1

The Moms Guide to Understanding the Best Supplements and Nutrients for A Healthy Growing Baby

MIA ANGELS

By reading this document, the reader agrees that under no circumstances is the author responsible for any losses, direct or indirect, which are incurred as a result of the use of information contained within this document, including, but not limited to, —errors, omissions, or inaccuracies.

Table of Contents

Introduction

Pregnancy is one of the most beautiful stages in a woman's life. Most of the time, you are not told about what you will need to live through during your pregnancy. You are also not warned about the many changes that you will need to make to your lifestyle. Truth be told, pregnancy is not a fairytale, and it is important that you are prepared for a few things. There are some that you will be aware about, but there are some things that are often concealed from you, and it is important that you know what these things are.

Pregnancy will change the way you lead your life, and it will change you forever. You will need to change the way you eat, and remember that you are eating for two people. Now when most women hear this, they believe that they need to double their food intake. What they do not realize is that they need to focus on what they are eating and not how much food they are eating. You should ensure that you consume food that is nutritious and healthy for you and your baby.

If you have recently found out that you are pregnant, you will have been given enough advice on what food you should eat and what you shouldn't. The amount of information thrown at you may have overwhelmed you. This book will put you at ease. You will learn everything you need to know about nutrition and the type of food you should eat.

Over the course of the book, you will learn more about why it is important for you to eat well, and the different nutrients you will need to consume regularly. You will also gather information on the different types of food you are allowed to eat and those that you must avoid. Remember that you should avoid some foods at all costs to keep your baby safe. You will also be given a few tips that will help you maintain your weight and obtain the required nutrition. It is important for you to remember that you will be consuming food for two people, and you should increase your intake of some nutrients to promote your health and your baby's health.

Thank you for purchasing the book. I hope the information in the book will help you learn more about how to stay healthy during your pregnancy.

Chapter One: Importance of Food During Pregnancy

It is always important to consider what type of food you are eating during your pregnancy, and not look at the quantity. Studies show that women only need to consume 450 extra calories during their pregnancy, and this is only when the baby starts to grow quickly. You can easily consume these extra calories by consuming a bowl of cereal with full-fat milk. Even if you increase your food intake, you should ensure that you consume only nutritious food since this will help with the development and growth of your baby.

Eating Well When You're Pregnant

Most women are surprised to note that they have gained 35 pounds during their pregnancy, especially when a baby weighs only a quarter of that. The pounds that you gain will add up in the following manner, but this will vary from one woman to another.

- 7.5 pounds: The weight of your baby
- 7 pounds: The stored fat, protein and other macro and micro nutrients
- 4 pounds: The extra blood
- 4 pounds: The extra fluids in the body
- 2 pounds: The large breasts
- 2 pounds: Your uterus enlarging
- 2 pounds: The amniotic fluid that surrounds your baby
- 1.5 pounds: The placenta in the womb

It is true that the pattern of weight gain will vary from one woman to another during their pregnancy. There are some women who will gain less weight if they were already heavy before they were pregnant, while there are others who will weigh a lot more if they have triplets or twins. You may also gain very little weight if you were underweight before your pregnancy. It is okay to gain weight, but it is important to know why you have gained that weight. The main source of nourishment for your baby is the food that you consume during your pregnancy. It was only recently that people began to understand that there is a very strong link between the food that you consume and the health of your baby. It is for this reason that doctors say that you should never drink alcohol, even if it is a small amount, during your pregnancy.

It is important for you to remember that the extra food that you consume should not only be calories. The food should be nutritious. For instance, calcium will help to keep your bones and teeth strong, and when you consume extra calcium you will be strengthening your baby's bones. The same can be said about all the food that you eat.

Nutrition for Expectant Moms

A balanced diet will include carbohydrates, proteins, vitamins, fats, minerals and at least two liters of water. You can use the guidelines provided by the US government to determine the number of servings of food that you should consume every day. It is always a good idea to consume different types of food since that will help you stay healthy.

Every packet of food that you purchase will have a food label that will tell you about the different types of nutrients in that food. The recommended daily allowance or RDA that is present on the food label will tell you what quantity of each nutrient you should consume every day. The RDA for most nutrients is usually high when you are pregnant.

Let us look at some nutrients that you should consume, and the food that contain those nutrients:

- Protein: This nutrient is essential for blood production and cell growth. The best sources of food for this nutrient are poultry, beans, egg whites, peanut butter, lean meat, fish and tofu.

- Carbohydrates: This nutrient is essential for the production of energy. The best sources of food for this nutrient are cereals, potatoes, rice, breads, fruit, vegetables and pasta.

- Calcium: This nutrient is essential to maintain the strength of teeth and bones, for muscle contraction and nerve function. The best sources of food for this nutrient are cheese, milk, sardines, salmon, yogurt and spinach.

- Iron: This nutrient is essential for the production of red blood cells to prevent anemia. The best sources of food for this nutrient are spinach, lean red meat, whole-grain and iron-fortified cereals and breads.

- Vitamin A: This nutrient is essential to maintain good eyesight, aid in the growth of bones and to maintain healthy skin. The best sources of food for this nutrient are dark leafy greens, carrots and sweet potatoes.

- Vitamin C: This nutrient is essential to maintain healthy teeth and gums. It also improves the body's ability to absorb iron. The best sources of food for this nutrient are broccoli, citrus fruit, fortified juices and tomatoes.

- Vitamin B6: This nutrient improves the body's ability to effectively use carbohydrates, fats and protein. The best sources of food for this nutrient are whole-grain cereals, pork, banana and ham.

- Vitamin B12: This nutrient is used to maintain and improve the functioning of the nervous system. The best sources of food for this nutrient are milk, poultry, fish and meat.

- Vitamin D: This nutrient helps to improve the body's ability to absorb calcium. The best sources of food for this nutrient are dairy products, breads, cereals and fortified milk.

- Folic Acid: The benefits of this nutrient have been discussed in detail in the next chapter. The best sources of food for this nutrient are dark yellow fruit, beans, nuts, green leafy vegetables and peas.

- Fat: This nutrient is stored as energy in the body. The sources of food for this nutrient are nuts, meat, peanut butter, whole-milk products, vegetable oils and margarine.

Every scientist is aware that your baby's health is dependent on the food that you consume. You should take care of your diet even before you are pregnant. For instance, studies show that folic acid is one of the only nutrients that can help to reduce the risk of developing neural tube defects during the early development stages of the fetus. It is for this reason that it is important that you consume this mineral in large quantities before your pregnancy and during the first few weeks of your pregnancy.

Doctors always suggest that women should take supplements for folic acids during their pregnancy, especially for the first four weeks. If you are considering pregnancy, you should speak to your doctor about your intake of folic acid. Another important nutrient that you should consider is calcium. This mineral is essential for the development and growth of your baby. Since your baby will absorb the calcium from the food that you contain, you should increase your intake to prevent any loss of calcium from your bones. Your doctor will also give you some prenatal vitamins that will have more folic acid and calcium.

The best sources of calcium are dairy products and milk. If you are lactose intolerant or are nauseous when you drink milk or consume dairy products, you can request your doctor to prescribe some calcium supplements. You are lactose intolerant if you develop gas, have bloating around your stomach and have diarrhea when you eat milk products or drink milk. You can either use lactose-free milk products or take a lactase capsule to help you digest the lactose. Other foods that are rich in calcium are salmon with bones, sardines, broccoli, tofu, calcium-fortified juices and spinach.

It is recommended that you do not begin a vegan diet during your pregnancy. If you were always a vegetarian or a vegan, you can continue this diet during your pregnancy, but you will need to be careful about the food that you eat. It will be difficult to obtain the right nutrition when you do not consume chicken, fish, eggs, milk and cheese. You will need to take protein supplements and Vitamin D and Vitamin B12 supplements.

You should consult a physician and a nutritionist during your pregnancy to ensure that you and your baby receive the required nutrition.

Food Cravings During Pregnancy

You probably know many women who have had cravings during their pregnancy, and you may have had some cravings yourself. There are some theories that state that a woman's craving for a specific type of food during pregnancy will indicate that the woman's body lacks the nutrients present in that food. This is definitely not a correct assumption, and doctors and researchers are still unsure why women have these cravings.

During their pregnancy, some women crave fruit, comfort food like cereals, mashed potatoes and toasted bread, chocolates and spicy food. Some women also crave cornstarch, clay and other non-food items, and this type of eating is called pica. If you consume things that are not food, you will endanger yourself and your baby. If you find yourself having some non-food cravings, you should consult your doctor immediately.

It is okay to give into your cravings if you ensure that you consume nutritious food in your other meals. You will find yourself craving for different types of food only during the first few months of your pregnancy.

Food and Drinks to Avoid While Pregnant

You should never consume alcohol during your pregnancy because it is not safe for you or your baby. You should also check with your doctor before you consume any herbal products or take any vitamin supplements since they can harm the development and growth of the fetus. There are some doctors who say that you can consume two cups of coffee, soda or tea every day since this amount of caffeine will not harm you or your baby. That said, it is wise to avoid caffeine altogether if you can since caffeine can lead to numerous problems and miscarriage. Try to switch to decaffeinated products or limit your intake of caffeine. We will look at some of the different foods that you should avoid in the last chapter of the book.

Managing Some Common Problems

Constipation

Pregnant women often have constipation because of the iron that is present in the prenatal vitamins. There are numerous other factors that can cause constipation too. It is for this reason that you should eat more fiber during your pregnancy. Try to consume at least thirty grams of fiber every day. The best sources for fiber are cereals, whole-grain breads, muffins, fruit and vegetables.

There are some people who use substitutes in the form of drinks or tablets, but it is important that you check with your doctor before you consume these products. You should avoid using laxatives unless your doctor specifically asks you to consume them. You should also avoid drinking castor oil since it will affect your body's ability to absorb the required vitamins and minerals from the food you consume.

If you have constipation regularly, you should ask your doctor for a stool softener. You should ensure that you drink a lot of water and increase your intake of fiber. If you do not do this, you will make the constipation worse. If you have the energy, you should try to exercise since this helps to avoid constipation. Drink enough water during the day. Always drink two glasses of water after your meal to make it easier for you to move the food through the digestive system. You can also consume broth, soups or tea.

Gas

Food like spinach, broccoli, fried foods and cauliflower can give some women gas or heartburn during their pregnancy. If you feel that this happens to you, you should consume a diet where you consume substitutes for these foods. You should also try to avoid carbonated drinks since they can cause heartburn and gas.

Nausea

Most women are nauseated during the first trimester. So, instead of avoiding food, you should try to consume small portions of food that is bland, like crackers or toast. You can also consume food that is made with ginger. Let us look at a few tips that will help you combat nausea.

- Never take your prenatal vitamins on an empty stomach. It is recommended that you consume these vitamins before you go to bed if you have eaten a snack.
- Try to consume a small snack whenever you wake up in the morning to use the washroom.
- Try to suck on hard candy.

Chapter Two: Important Nutrients

Now that you know why it is important to focus on the type of food you are eating, let us look at some of the macronutrients and micronutrients that you should consume during your pregnancy.

Macronutrients

Energy

The amount of energy you consume will determine the amount of weight you gain during your pregnancy. It is important to remember that you will need to eat the required amount of energy during your pregnancy to ensure that you supply your body with the usual amount and also support the growth and development of the fetus. The extra energy that you consume will help in the growth and development of existing tissue and new tissue. You will not find that you need more energy during the first trimester of your pregnancy. It is only from the second trimester that you will need more energy. The growth of the tissue in the mother and the fetus is more from the second trimester. That said, the energy that a pregnant woman needs during her pregnancy is dependent on many other factors like the body mass index (BMI) before pregnancy, the metabolic rate and the physical activity levels. Therefore, you should tailor your need for energy depending on your body.

The global estimate suggests that pregnant women need to consume at least 9260 kJ of energy per day. You must ensure that you provide your body with the required amount of energy to reduce the risk of miscarriages, premature birth and stillbirth. When you provide your body with less energy, your weight will automatically reduce. There is, however, very little research to determine whether the consumption of energy can be restricted.

A study was conducted on 384 subjects, and an analysis was made based on three trials. This study reported that women who gained too much weight during pregnancy or were overweight before pregnancy can reduce their consumption of energy to obtain their ideal gestational weight. Two of these trials, however, reported that any reduction in the consumption of energy could have adverse effects on the baby's birth weight. It is important to prevent maternal obesity, but it is also important to reduce the risk of any complications during birth. Given that there is very little evidence, it is advised that pregnant women do not reduce the consumption of energy.

Protein

Protein is a macronutrient that is required for both structural and functional biological roles. The primary source of protein across the globe is from plant-based foods like grains, nuts and legumes, followed by animal-based foods and dairy. There are some alternative sources for protein like bacteria, fungi and algae. These are known as micro proteins. The quality of protein is determined based on its capacity to meet the requirement of amino acids and nitrogen that are necessary for maintenance, growth and repair and its digestibility. Animal protein is termed as a complete protein since it provides the required quantity of nitrogen and indispensable amino acids. The plant-based proteins are incomplete proteins since they will be deficient in at least one protein like threonine or lysine.

Based on the current recommendations by the US Government, the consumption of at least 16.1% protein of the total energy is adequate for pregnant women. There will be some adjustments that your body makes in the protein metabolism during the first few weeks of pregnancy. This is done to maintain homeostasis in the mother's body while accommodating the needs and demands of the fetus. Studies show that protein is synthesized in large quantities from the second trimester to cater to the fetus' needs. If you are well nourished, these changes will help to conserve nitrogen and protein, and also promote the accumulation of protein to ensure that the fetus obtains the required nutrition.

Fiber, Glycemic Index and Glycemic Load

You can obtain carbohydrates from numerous sources, and each of these foods has a different digestion rate. Therefore, the effect of these foods will affect the insulin levels and the blood glucose levels differently. The glycemic index for each source will quantify your body's response that is induced by the carbohydrates. Foods like white bread, potatoes and rice have a high glycemic index, and they cause a sharp increase in the blood glucose levels when consumed. The levels also decline rapidly once the food has been digested. Foods like dairy products and fruit have a low glycemic index, and the carbohydrates in these foods are digested slowly. This results in a low response to glucose. The glycemic load will look at both the quantity of carbohydrates and the glycemic index of the food. You can calculate the glycemic load in food by multiplying the carbohydrate content with the glycemic index.

The dietary fiber is the plant-based carbohydrate that we consume. These carbohydrates cannot be digested by the human digestive system. Dietary fiber includes starch resistant fiber that is obtained from cooked rice and potato, and soluble fiber, which is obtained from vegetables, fruit and legumes. Doctors and researchers advise women to consume food with a low glycemic index and glycemic load, and food that is rich in fiber to modulate and maintain the blood glucose levels, reduce constipation and also reduce the cholesterol levels in blood.

Fatty Acids

Down of the essential fatty acids are the short-chain fatty acids including alpha-linoleic and linoleic acids, and the long-chain derivatives including Docosahexaenoic acid (DHA), Eicosapentaenoic acid (EPA) and Arachidonic acid (AA). These fatty acids are required for the formation of tissues and are used to build the cell membranes. Some foods that are rich in these fatty acids include oily fish like salmon and mackerel and some fish oil supplements. The concentration of these fats decreases in the body during pregnancy by at least 40%. Therefore, it is important that a woman increase her intake of fatty acids, especially the long-chain fatty acids during pregnancy. This is the only way that the mother can meet the dietary requirements of her body and the fetus. DHA can help to develop the retina and brain in the fetus. EPA can help to reduce the production of thromboxane A2. If you are unable to consume the required quantity of Vitamin D through your diet, you should ask your doctor to suggest some supplements.

Micronutrients in Pregnancy

Folate

Folate is present in yeast extract, citrus fruit like oranges and leafy green vegetables. It is a water-soluble vitamin. There are some breakfast cereals and bread that are fortified with folic acid, which is the more stable and synthetic form of folate. This vitamin acts as a coenzyme during the methylation cycles in the body, and helps to transfer carbon through the body. It is integral for the synthesis of neurotransmitters and DNA. This vitamin is also used in the synthesis of proteins, multiplication of cells and the metabolism of amino acids. This makes it important for pregnant women to increase their intake of folate during the first few weeks of pregnancy since the fetus will grow rapidly because of cell division and growth of tissues. Deficiency of folate will result in the accumulation of homocysteine. This will increase the risk of preeclampsia and anomalies or abnormalities in the fetus.

It is important to consume folic acid during the first few weeks of pregnancy to reduce the risk of developing neural tube defects. The neural tube is developed in the first few weeks of pregnancy, and it is important to take folic acid supplements to aid in the growth of the tube.

Vitamin A

Vitamin A can be derived from provitamin carotenoids and preformed retinoids. Retinoids, like retinoic acid and retinal acid, can be obtained from different animal sources including fish liver oil, liver, dairy and eggs. Carotenoids like beta-carotene can be obtained from numerous plants like yellow or dark vegetables like sweet potatoes, carrots and kale. These compounds are converted into Vitamin A by the body, and stored in the liver. Some physiological functions of Vitamin A are bone metabolism, growth, gene transcription and immune function. This vitamin enhances the antioxidant activities in the body. Women are advised to consume more vitamin A during pregnancy since this vitamin will be used to support the growth of the fetus and maintain the tissues. If you are unable to obtain the required intake of Vitamin A, you can consume supplements. The effects of vitamin A on the body during pregnancy vary, and further research needs to be conducted to understand this better. It is, however, important that women monitor the levels of Vitamin A in their body to ensure that the vitamin is not being accumulated in the liver leading to toxicity.

Vitamin B_1 (Thiamine), Vitamin B_3 (Niacin), Vitamin B_6 (Pyridoxine), Vitamin B_2 (Riboflavin), and Vitamin B_{12} (Cyanocobalamin)

Vitamin B is a complex vitamin, and it includes B_1 (Thiamine), B_3 (Niacin), B_6 (Pyridoxine), B_2 (Riboflavin), and B_{12} (Cyanocobalamin). These vitamins are water-soluble and are used by the body for the production of energy in cells. It is also required for the metabolism of fats, carbohydrates and protein. These vitamins also act as coenzymes, and is used in numerous metabolic pathways for the formation of blood cells and also in the generation of energy. Vitamin B12 works with Folate to generate methionine from homocysteine. This process is required for the methylation of neurotransmitters, phospholipids, proteins, DNA and RNA. A deficiency in these vitamins will negatively impact the growth of cells and the growth of nerve tissues. Women are advised to take prenatal vitamins during pregnancy, and these vitamins contain Vitamin B_1 (Vitamin B.

Vitamin B-complex can be found in large quantities in fortified cereals, leafy green vegetables, legumes and animal products including dairy products, fish, poultry and meat. Pregnant women are required to increase their intake of vitamin B since there is an increase in the protein and energy required by the body.

Vitamin C and E

Vitamin E and Vitamin C are fat-soluble and water-soluble vitamins. Vitamin E is a group of eight compounds that are obtained from plants, of which four compounds are tocotienols, namely alpha, beta, gamma and delta, and four tocopherols, namely alpha, beta, gamma and delta. The alpha-tocopherol is a biologically active compound. Vitamin C can be found in a variety of fruit and vegetables like citrus fruit, broccoli, tomatoes and guava. Vitamin E can be found in vegetable oils, wheat germ oil, some leafy vegetables and nuts. Vitamins C and E increase the formation of radicals in the body, which help to reduce oxidative stress. These vitamins also improve the immune system. Vitamin C also increases the synthesis of collagen. This compound is one of the primary components of connective tissues, and enhances the body's ability to absorb iron, thereby reducing iron deficiency and preventing megaloblastic anemia.

During pregnancy, the body transports the vitamin C consumed into the placenta. This reduces the amount of Vitamin C in the mother's body thereby increasing the daily intake to 85 milligrams a day.

Vitamin D

Vitamin D is an essential nutrient required to maintain the integrity of bones and also maintain calcium homeostasis in the body. Vitamin D is also required for the performance of some extra skeletal functions including its role in reducing inflammation, improving the function of the immune system, angiogenesis and the metabolism of glucose. It is also used in the regulation of gene expression and transcription. The body absorbs Vitamin D when it is exposed to the sun. You can also obtain Vitamin D from few foods like fortified dairy products and oily fish. If you do not meet the required intake of Vitamin D, you can take some supplements in the form of ergocalciferol (vitamin D2) and cholecalciferol (vitamin D3).

When Vitamin D is synthesized or ingested, it is first broken down in the liver to form the Vitamin hydroxyvitamin D (25(OH) D). This form of the vitamin is what can be circulated. The quantity of this form of the vitamin in the body is used to determine if there is a deficiency or not. Vitamin D is also broken down in the kidneys to create the active form of the vitamin, 1,25-dihydroxyvitamin D (1,25(OH) 2D3).

The deficiency of Vitamin D can be attributed to pigmented skin, lack of exposure to sunlight because of a sedentary lifestyle, the use of protective clothing or sunscreen and a low intake of fortified foods. It is important to control your intake of Vitamin D and also to prevent a deficiency especially during pregnancy.

Calcium

Calcium is one of the most essential nutrients to strengthen bones. It is also an important component that is found in the membranes around the cells. This mineral is used in numerous biological processes including muscle contractions, hormone homeostasis, signal transduction and enzyme homeostasis. It is also important to improve the function of neurons. Some of the best sources of calcium are dairy products and milk, but this mineral can also be obtained from fortified foods like dairy alternatives and flour, leafy green vegetables and nuts.

During pregnancy, the mother's body will automatically transfer the calcium from the placenta into the fetus. It is for this reason that the mother's need for calcium increases, especially during the third trimester. Calcium is used efficiently during pregnancy because of the changes made to the mother's physiology. During pregnancy, a woman's body will absorb more calcium because of the hormonal changes in the body. The kidneys will also retain calcium in their tubules during pregnancy. A woman can meet the required intake of calcium through her diet alone, but supplements can be taken to ensure that there is a balance in the calcium levels in the woman's body.

Calcium deficiency can lead to paresthesia, tetanus, tremors, muscle cramps and osteopenia. It can also lead to delayed growth in the fetus, poor mineralization in the bones and LBW. Studies show that women who consume very little calcium may develop hypertensive disorders during pregnancy.

Iodine

Iron is one of the many nutrients that aids in regulating metabolism, growth and development through the synthesis of the triiodothyronine (T3) and thyroxine (T4) hormones. This nutrient is obtained from fortified salt, but can also be sourced from various seafood and kelp. Iodine can also be obtained from plant and dairy products that have been sourced from iodine-fortified animal feed or sowed in iodine-rich soil. The hormonal alterations and metabolic demands during pregnancy increase the need for iodine. The demands increase because the production of the thyroid hormone during the first trimester increases by 50% and the excretion of iodine also increases by 50%. It is only later during the gestation period that the iodine is passed through the placenta to the fetus.

The thyroid hormones in the mother and the fetus regulate some of the key development processes. The hormones regulate the development of the nervous system in the fetus, and also aid in the formation of the myelination and synapses, and the growth of the nerve cells. You will only need to consume small quantities of iodine to prevent deficiency. However, iodine deficiency disorders are the main reason behind cognitive impairments in the fetus. Other consequences of iodine deficiencies are lower Intelligent Quotient (IQ) in children, stillbirth, miscarriage and fetal goiter.

Iron

Iron is essential for the synthesis of myoglobin and hemoglobin in the blood. It is a vital nutrient used for numerous cellular functions including respiration, oxygen transport, Gene regulation, growth and the functioning of those enzymes that are made up of iron. It is for this reason that it is necessary that the right quantity of iron is stored in the body to ensure homeostasis. Having said that, iron deficiency is one of the most common deficiencies across the world. Pregnant women have low iron content in their body because they do not consume the right food to improve the body's ability to absorb iron. They may also have iron deficiency if they are affected by any parasites. It is for this reason that it is important to increase your intake of plant-based foods like green leafy vegetables. These vegetables contain non-heam iron used in different bodily functions. That said, the body absorbs the heam iron from animal meat and fish easily, and it is because of this that these products are the main source of iron for mammals.

During pregnancy, the need for iron increases to 7.5 milligrams a day, although it is hard to determine the amount required during the third trimester. Iron is needed to fulfill the needs of the fetus, for the expansion of the erythrocyte mass in the mother and to compensate for the loss of iron. Since the iron required during pregnancy increases during pregnancy, the chances of developing an iron deficiency also increase. A study conducted by WHO concluded that close to 38.2% pregnant women have an iron deficiency and are anemic.

Anemia and iron deficiency are known to increase the risk of premature birth, SGA or LBW infants, lower immunity against diseases and infection, impaired bodily functions in the mother and abnormal development of cognitive function and psychomotor development in the fetus.

Zinc

Zinc is one of the most important nutrients that one should consume because it contains over 200 enzymes and is a structural component in numerous hormones, proteins and nucleotides. This mineral has the most important biochemical functions since it aids in the synthesis of proteins and also helps to break down nucleic acids in the human body. This mineral also aids in gene expression, cellular division, wound healing, immune and neurological function, antioxidant defenses and vision.

Zinc can be found in different types of food, but large quantities of this mineral are found in seafood, nuts, milk and meat. Diets that are rich in fiber will reduce the quantity of zinc found in the body. The amount of zinc present in the body can be measured by checking the levels of zinc in the plasma or serum. The values will vary depending on the sex, age, physiological factors like infection or stress and the time of day. Due to this it becomes difficult for people to accurately determine whether they are deficient. It is, however, estimated that close to 82 percent of pregnant women are deficient in zinc. Doctors recommend that pregnant women consume at least fifteen milligrams of zinc from the second trimester.

Studies show that close to half a million child and maternal deaths a year occur due to deficiency in zinc, and this is especially true for developing countries. Deficiency in zinc has been associated with prolonged labor, intrauterine growth retardation, pregnancy-induced hypertension, LBW, impaired immunity and pre-term and post-term births. If your body has trouble with absorbing zinc, it can lead to a miscarriage or congenital malfunctions.

Two separate studies were conducted to understand the effects of zinc during pregnancy. These studies reported that the use of zinc supplements during pregnancy helped to reduce the risk of premature birth by at least fourteen percent. That said, there was no effect of these supplements on the neonatal mortality, birth weight and hypertensive disorders. Doctors believe that zinc helps to reduce the risk of premature birth by reducing the risk of infections during pregnancy.

Chapter Three: Healthy Foods Equals Healthy Baby

As mentioned earlier, it is important to ensure that you maintain your health during pregnancy. It is during this time that you will need to provide your body with additional vitamins, minerals and nutrients. As mentioned earlier, you will need to increase your intake of calories by 450, but will also need to focus on the nutrition. If you consume food that is not nutritious, it will impact the development of the baby. Excess weight gain and poor eating habits can increase the risk of complications during birth and gestational diabetes. In simple terms, if you choose to consume nutritious food, you can ensure the health of your baby and yourself. It will also make it very easy for you to lose all the weight you put on during pregnancy once you give birth. This chapter lists some of the best foods that you should consume during your pregnancy.

Dairy Products

It is important for you to increase your intake of calcium and protein during pregnancy to ensure that you meet the needs of your baby. There are two high-quality proteins that are found in dairy products – whey and casein. Dairy is also one of the best sources of calcium, and it provides large quantities of magnesium, Vitamin B, zinc and phosphorous. Doctors advise pregnant women to consume yogurt, especially Greek yogurt since that contains more protein and calcium when compared to other dairy products. There are some types of yogurt that also contain probiotic bacteria that aid in digestion. If you are lactose intolerant, you may be able to tolerate probiotic yogurt. You can also take some probiotic supplements to reduce the risk of any complications that may arise during pregnancy like vaginal infections, gestational diabetes, preeclampsia and allergies.

Legumes

Legumes are a group of food that includes peas, lentils, chickpeas, peanuts, beans and soybeans. Legumes are rich in protein, folate, calcium and iron, and they are the best source of fiber. Your body needs each of these nutrients in large quantities during pregnancy. Folate is an essential vitamin that helps to maintain the health of both the fetus and the mother. Unfortunately, most women do not consume the required quantity of folate during their pregnancy, which can lead to low birth weight and neural tube defects. It is for this reason that you should increase your intake of folate during the first trimester. Insufficient folate can also impact your child's immune system, which can render him or her defenseless to some diseases and infections. Legumes are rich in folate, and one serving of lentils provides at least ninety percent of the required intake of folate.

Sweet Potatoes

Sweet potatoes are rich in a plant compound called beta-carotene. This compound helps to convert the vitamin A in the human body into a useable form. This vitamin aids in the development and growth of the tissues and cells in the fetus, and is extremely important for the development of the fetus. Doctors recommend that pregnant women should increase their intake of Vitamin A by at least 40 percent. That said, they are also advised to reduce their intake of Vitamin A from animal-based sources since this can lead to toxicity in the body. Sweet potatoes are rich in beta-carotene, and one cup of cooked sweet potato a day is enough to fulfill the daily requirement of beat-carotene. Sweet potatoes also contain fiber. This nutrient will reduce the spikes in blood sugar, improve digestion, improve mobility and satiate your hunger.

Salmon

Salmon is one of the best sources of omega-3 fatty acids, and most people, especially pregnant women, do not consume the required amount of omega-3 fatty acids through their diet. The long chain Omega-3 fatty acids like EPA and DHA are essential during pregnancy, and these acids are found in large quantities in seafood. They help in the growth and development of your fetus's eyes and brain. That said, women are advised to limit their intake of seafood to twice a week or lesser depending on the Mercury content in the fish. Since Mercury is a fatal compound, most women avoid fish altogether because they worry about their baby. This limits their intake of Omega-3 fatty acids. Studies show that Willem who consume at least two meals of low-mercury and fatty-fish consume the required amount of omega-3 fatty acids. This helps to increase the levels of EPA and DHA in the blood. Salmon is one of the very few natural sources of Vitamin D, and this is a vitamin that is lacking in most people's diet. This vitamin endures the health of your bones, improves the function of the immune system and aids numerous processes that take place in the human body.

Eggs

Eggs are the best food to consume since they contain every nutrient that your body needs. One large egg is rich is high-quality fat and protein, and adds 77 calories to your diet. This food is also rich in numerous vitamins and minerals. Eggs are the best source of choline, and this mineral is required for a variety of processes in the human body, especially in the development of the brain. A survey conducted in the US showed that close to ninety percent of the people consumed very little choline. If you eat less choline, you will harm your fetus. A low intake can lead to decreased function in the brain of the fetus and also increase the risk of developing neural tube defects. One egg contains at least 113 milligrams of choline, and this covers at least twenty-five percent of the required intake.

Dark, Leafy Greens and Broccoli

Dark, leafy greens, like spinach and kale, and broccoli are rich in nutrients that every pregnant woman should consume. These nutrients include vitamin K, vitamin C, vitamin A, potassium, folate, iron and fiber. Leafy greens and broccoli have antioxidants and plant compounds that aid in digestion and improve the immune system. Since these vegetables are rich in fiber, they will help to prevent constipation. As mentioned earlier, this is a problem that most pregnant women face. You can also reduce the risk of low birth weight by increasing your intake of leafy vegetables.

Lean Meat

Pork, chicken and beef are the best sources of lean protein. Pork and beef are rich in choline, vitamin B and iron, which are the nutrients that are required in abundance during pregnancy. Red blood cells require iron to increase the hemoglobin content. Hemoglobin is used to pass oxygen to every cell in your body. Since the blood volume increases during pregnancy, it is important for women to increase their intake of iron especially during the third trimester. Iron deficiency during the first trimester can increase the risk of low birth weight and premature delivery. Many women do not like meat during their pregnancy, and this makes it hard for them to consume the required amount of iron through their diet alone. For those who can eat meat, you should consume at least one serving of red meat on alternate days to increase the amount of iron that you acquire through your diet. The consumption of foods rich in vitamin C will help to improve your body's ability to absorb iron.

Fish Liver Oil

Fish liver oil is often extracted from the codfish. The oil is taken from the oily liver. This oil is rich in long chain omega-3 fatty acids like DHA and EPA. These are essential for the development of the eye and brain. Fish liver oil is rich in Vitamin D, and most people do not get enough of this vitamin. If you do not consume seafood, you will need to consume a vitamin D or Omega-3 supplement. Low vitamin D increases the risk of preeclampsia which is a complication today is potentially dangerous. This complication is characterized by the swelling of feet and hands, protein in the urine and high blood pressure. When you consume cod liver oil during the first few weeks of pregnancy, you can ensure that your baby has a high birth weight. One serving of this oil can help you meet your daily intake requirement of vitamin A, Vitamin D and omega-3 fatty acids. You should, however, ensure that you do not consume too much since that will lead to vitamin A toxicity in your body.

Berries

Berries are rich in Vitamin C, antioxidants and fiber, and are packed with healthy carbs and water. Vitamin C improves your body's ability to absorb iron, and this vitamin is also essential to improve the functioning of the immune system and maintain skin health. Berries do not cause any spikes in the blood sugar levels because they have a very low glycemic index. Since these fruits contain both fiber and water, they are a great snack, and they are nutritious and have a low number of calories.

Whole Grains

It is important for women to consume whole grains during their pregnancy since this helps them increase their intake of calories. Whole grains are rich in plant compounds, fiber and vitamins when compared to refined grains. Quinoa and oats contain a good amount of protein, and this nutrient is essential to consume during pregnancy since it helps to maintain and repair the tissues in the body. Whole grains are also rich in magnesium, Vitamin B and fiber.

Avocados

Avocados are probably the only fruit that is rich in monosaturated fatty acids. This fruit is also rich in Vitamin K, Vitamin B, folate, Vitamin E, Vitamin C, copper, potassium and fiber. Since avocados are rich in potassium, healthy fats and folate, doctors and nutritionists advise women to consume avocados. The healthy fats help to build the brain, tissues and the skin of your fetus, and the folate reduces the risk of developing neural tube defects. One of the side effects of pregnancy is leg cramps, and potassium helps to relieve these cramps.

Dried Fruit

Dried fruit are rich in various vitamins, minerals and fiber, and high in calories. There is no difference between fresh fruit and dry fruit except for the fact that the latter has no water and is smaller in size. Therefore, you will consume the required intake of numerous vitamins and minerals including iron, potassium and folate when you consume one serving of dried fruit. Prunes are rich in Vitamin K, sorbitol, fiber and potassium, and they are natural laxatives. If you have constipation, you should consume at least one serving of this fruit every day. Dates are rich in potassium, plant compounds, fiber and iron, and it is important for women to consume dates regularly during the first and third trimesters since this will help to reduce the need for induced labor and also help to facilitate in the dilation of the cervix. Dried fruit also contains large quantities of natural sugar, and it is for this reason that you avoid the consumption of the candied dried fruit. Dried fruit does help to increase your intake of nutrients and calories, but doctors recommend that women consume only one serving of dried fruit per day during their pregnancy.

Water

The volume of blood will increase by 50 ounces during pregnancy, and it is important that you stay hydrated during your pregnancy. If you do not watch your intake of water, you will soon be dehydrated because your baby will get everything that he or she needs from you. Some symptoms of mild dehydration are anxiety, headaches, bad mood, reduced memory and tiredness. When you increase your intake of water, you can reduce the risk of urinary tract infections and also help to relieve constipation. These are common issues that women have during pregnancy. Women are advised to drink at least two liters of water every day during their pregnancy, but the amount varies for each individual. You should also bear in mind that you do get water from food and beverages like coffee, tea, vegetables and fruit. It is important that you drink water whenever you are thirsty, and drink the required amount of water to quench your thirst.

Chapter Four: Unhealthy Foods Equals Unhealthy Baby

It is a known fact that the most sensitive period or time in a woman's life is pregnancy, and it is important that women consume a healthy diet during that time. It is also important for women who are trying to get pregnant to consume a healthy diet. This chapter lists different foods that women should avoid during their pregnancy.

High-Mercury Fish

Mercury is one of the most toxic elements, and this element is often found in polluted water. There is no amount of Mercury that is considered safe. Large quantities of mercury are toxic to the kidneys, nervous system and immune system. Mercury can also lead to some developmental issues in children. Most marine fish have large amounts of mercury in their body, and it is for this reason that women are advised to consume only one or two servings of high-mercury fish per month during their pregnancy. Some fish that have high-mercury are:

- Tuna, especially albacore tuna
- Swordfish
- King mackerel
- Shark

It is, however, important for you to understand that every marine fish does not have too much mercury. It is only some types that have large quantities of mercury in their body. It is essential that you consume low-mercury fish during your pregnancy, and it is healthy to consume one serving of this fish at least twice a week.

Raw or Undercooked Fish

Raw fish can lead to several infections that can be parasitic, bacterial or viral like Salmonella, Vibrio, Listeria and norovirus. A few of these infections only affect the mother and often leave her weak and dehydrated. Some infections can pass on to the fetus and lead to serious, and sometimes fatal, consequences. Most women are vulnerable to the Listeria bacteria during their pregnancy. Studies show that pregnant women are twenty percent more likely to develop an infection caused by Listeria when compared to the general population. Listeria can be found in soil, polluted water and on contaminated fruit and vegetables. Raw fish is often infected by Listeria during smoking and drying. Mothers may not show any symptoms if they are affected by Listeria, but these bacteria will pass to the fetus through the placenta. This can lead to miscarriage, stillbirth, premature delivery and other health issues. It is for this reason that women are advised to avoid raw fish during their pregnancy. This means that you cannot consume sushi ever.

Raw, Processed and Undercooked Meat

You will increase the risk of developing infections from several parasites and bacteria, like Listeria, Salmonella, E.coli and Toxoplasma, if you eat raw or undercooked meat. The bacteria and parasites can threaten the health of your baby. If you are infected by any of these parasites, the risk of developing severe neurological illnesses or stillbirth increases. The risk of developing intellectual disabilities, epilepsy and blindness also increases. Most of the bacteria in meat is present on the surface and can easily be washed off. There are times when these bacteria are present inside the fibers of the muscles. You can consume the sirloins, ribeye and tenderloins of lamb, veal and beef even if they are not cooked fully. It is important to remember that this holds good only for the meat that is uncut or whole. Cut meat including burgers, meat patties, pork, minced meat and poultry should always be consumed when they are cooked fully. Deli meat, lunchmeat and hot dogs also must be consumed when fully cooked, because bacteria or parasites can contaminate them during storage or processing. It is for this reason that women should always consume processed meat products only when they are steaming hot.

Raw Eggs

Most raw eggs are contaminated with salmonella. Only the mother shows any symptoms of being affected by salmonella, and these symptoms include vomiting, nausea, fever, diarrhea and stomach cramps. However, these infections could lead to premature birth, stillbirth and terrible cramps in the uterus. Let us look at some foods that contain raw eggs:

- Homemade ice cream
- Homemade mayonnaise
- Poached eggs
- Lightly scrambled eggs
- Hollandaise sauce
- Salad dressings
- Cake icings

Commercial products often contain pasteurized raw eggs, and it is for this reason that you can consume these products during your pregnancy. Having said that, it is important that you always read the label to ensure that the eggs are pasteurized. It is important that you cook eggs or eat only pasteurized eggs.

Organ Meat

Organ meat is rich in vitamin B12, copper, iron and Vitamin A. These vitamins and minerals are essential for the health of the baby and the mother. That said, you should avoid the consumption of too much organ meat since that will increase the quantity of Vitamin A leading to toxicity in the body. Increased consumption of organ meat will increase the levels of copper in the body. This will result in liver toxicity and birth defects. It is for this reason that it is important that pregnant women do not consume more than one serving of organ meat per week.

Caffeine

One of the commonly used psychoactive substances is caffeine, and this substance is found in tea, coffees, cocoa and soft drinks. Doctors recommend that pregnant women limit their caffeine intake to only two cups of coffee a day. The body absorbs caffeine very quickly, and this compound quickly moves into the placenta. The levels of caffeine can build up inside the fetus and the placenta since neither has the enzyme that can break caffeine down. A high intake of caffeine can increase the risk of low birth weight and can also restrict the growth of the fetus. Low birth weight is directly linked to chronic diabetes, like heart disease and Type II diabetes, and infant death.

Raw Sprouts

Raw sprouts like clover, alfalfa, mung bean sprouts and radish are often contaminated with salmonella. These bacteria thrive in humid environments, and they are impossible to remove from the plants. It is for this reason that women are advised against the consumption of raw sprouts. Having said that, sprouts once cooked are safe to consume.

Unwashed Produce

Most vegetables and fruit are contaminated with several parasites and bacteria, including listeria, toxoplasma, Salmonella and E.coli. These bacteria and parasites can be acquired during handling or from the soil. It is important to remember that vegetables and fruit can get contaminated at any time during harvest, storage, production, retail and transportation. Bacteria and parasites can harm both the baby and the mother. Toxoplasma is one of the most dangerous parasites that linger on vegetables and fruit. Most people who have invested toxoplasma do not show any symptoms, but there are a few people who do have a cold or the flu for more than a month. There are times when the fetus is infected with toxoplasma, but the symptoms, like intellectual disabilities and blindness, only appear later in life. Some babies may be born with serious brain or eye damage. So, when you are pregnant you should always rinse, peel and cook vegetables and fruit to reduce the risk of developing infections.

Unpasteurized Fruit Juice, Cheese and Milk

Unpasteurized and raw milk and cheese will contain some harmful bacteria including E.coli, Salmonella, Campylobacter and Listeria. The same can be said about unpasteurized juice since these juices can be contaminated easily. Any of these bacterial infections can lead to life-threatening consequences for your baby. Some of these bacterial are present in these foods, and they multiply due to contamination during storage or collection. One of the best ways to effectively kill these bacteria is through pasteurization. This process does not reduce the nutritional content of the products. It is for this reason that women are advised to drink pasteurized fruit juice, milk and cheese.

Alcohol

Doctors recommend that women should avoid alcohol during their pregnancy since alcohol increases the risk of stillbirth and miscarriage. A small amount of alcohol can severely affect the development of your baby's brain, and can lead to fetal alcohol syndrome. As a result of this syndrome, your baby can develop intellectual disabilities, facial deformities and heart defects. There are no studies that can prove that small amounts of alcohol during pregnancy do not harm the mother or baby.

Processed Junk Food

During your pregnancy, you will notice that you and your baby are growing at a rapid rate. It is for this reason that you need to increase your intake of healthy nutrients including iron, protein and folate. It is true that you will be eating for two, but you do not need to double your caloric intake. As mentioned earlier, you will only need to increase your caloric intake by 450 calories. During your pregnancy, you will need to consume food that is rich in nutrients to ensure that you fulfill the needs of your body and your baby's. Processed junk food does not have any nutrients and is rich in added fats, sugar and calories. Studies show that added sugar can increase the risk of developing numerous diseases like heart disease and Type II Diabetes. It is necessary that you gain weight during pregnancy, but this excess weight gain can lead to different diseases, like gestational diabetes, and complications in birth. It can also increase the risk of giving birth to an overweight child, which will lead to some long-term health issues.

Chapter Five: Some Important Tips

It is important to ensure that you consume the right food during pregnancy to ensure the health of your baby. As mentioned earlier, when you consume the right food, you can reduce the risk of any illnesses or diseases that your child may develop after birth.

Eating for Two During Pregnancy

You will need to make sure that you change your eating habits during your pregnancy regardless of whether you were preparing to become pregnant or were surprised by the pregnancy. Numerous women start their pregnancy with a deficiency in numerous nutrients that are important for a healthy pregnancy. It is important that you meet the daily requirement of nutrients during your pregnancy since you will be eating for you and your baby. Research suggests that it is important for you to change your eating habits during your pregnancy since the food you eat then will determine the well-being of your child while he or she is in the womb, at birth and beyond birth. Your lifestyle will either increase or decrease the risk of your child developing numerous conditions like heart diseases, obesity and diabetes.

Always Focus on Folic Acid

You will have read repeatedly how important it is for you to consume folic acid during your pregnancy. Folic acid is one of the best ways to improve your child's health. As mentioned earlier, it is important for you to consume folic acid during the first trimester to reduce the risk of developing neural tube defects. It is important that you increase your intake of folic acid by consuming supplements. You should also consume fortified bread, cereal, pasta and rice.

Understand That Multivitamins Have Different Effects During Pregnancy

A multivitamin does not only provide the required nutrients for the mother and the baby, but has many other benefits. Studies show that prenatal vitamins and multivitamin tablets help to reduce the risk of preeclampsia, which increases the quantity of protein in the urine and increases blood pressure, by at least 40 percent. Preeclampsia can lead to premature birth or stillbirth. You may find it difficult to swallow your multivitamin tablets during pregnancy since these pills contain large quantities of iron that can cause constipation. These pills are also big which makes it difficult to swallow them. If you find that you have trouble with prenatal vitamins you should let your doctor know since you are having some unwanted side effects. Ensure that you let your doctor know about all the supplements that you are taking.

Always Make the Calories Count

It will be slightly difficult to monitor your weight gain during the first trimester. There are a few women who lose weight during this time since they have a lot of nausea and queasiness. This will prevent them from eating or drinking. If you are constantly nauseous or vomit often, you should consult your doctor because you will become dehydrated. Morning sickness often dissipates after the first few weeks of pregnancy, but you may feel nauseous throughout your pregnancy. When your baby begins to grow, you will need to increase your intake of calories by consuming food that is rich in nutrients. It is true that you will be eating for two people, but this does not mean that you can overeat. As mentioned earlier in the book, you will need to consume only 300 additional calories during your pregnancy. This may sound like a lot of calories. It is certainly okay to splurge on some hot chocolate or eat comfort food when you have cravings. You can make the additional calories that you consume in the following manner:

- 16 ounces of full fat or 1% low fat milk

- 2 ounces of chicken
- 1 teaspoon of mayonnaise
- 2 – 4 slices of whole-wheat bread
- 4 ounces non-fat or full-fast yogurt with fruit
- 1 ounce whole grain cereal

Weighty Matters During Pregnancy

It is important for you to gain the recommended number of pounds during your pregnancy to reduce any complications during delivery or pregnancy. Your weight will determine the health of your baby. Women who have a normal weight before they are pregnant will gain at least 35 pounds during pregnancy, but the weight will vary if they are giving birth to twins. It is important for women who are underweight or overweight to either gain more weight or lose weight before they become pregnant. If you were overweight before you became pregnant, you must ensure that you do not diet during your pregnancy. You should work closely with your dietician to ensure that you maintain your weight during your pregnancy.

Rethink Your Fluids During Pregnancy

You should ensure that you drink at least ten glasses of fluid every day during your pregnancy. You can drink plain water if you do not want to drink juice or milk. You should ensure that you do not consume any alcohol during your pregnancy since it can lead to some physical and mental defects in the baby. In the third and fourth chapter of the book, you will gather information about the different types of fluids that you can and cannot drink during your pregnancy.

Conclusion

Thank you for purchasing the book.

Pregnancy is one of the most cherished times in a woman's life. Having said that, it is also one of the most sensitive periods in a woman's life because she will need to take care of herself and her child. You will, therefore, need to ensure that you consume the right food to improve your health and also aid in the growth and development of the fetus.

Over the course of the book, you will have gathered information about the different foods that you should consume during pregnancy and also the list of foods you should avoid. If you follow the instructions given in the book word for word, you can ensure that you and your baby are healthy.

Sources

https://www.webmd.com/baby/features/top-tips-pregnancy-nutrition#4

https://www.ncbi.nlm.nih.gov/pmc/articles/PMC6413112/

https://www.johnmuirhealth.com/health-education/health-wellness/pregnancy-breastfeeding/nutritional-needs-during-pregnancy.html

https://www.ncbi.nlm.nih.gov/pmc/articles/PMC5084016/

https://www.healthline.com/nutrition/11-foods-to-avoid-during-pregnancy

https://www.healthline.com/nutrition/13-foods-to-eat-when-pregnant

https://www.mayoclinic.org/healthy-lifestyle/pregnancy-week-by-week/in-depth/pregnancy-nutrition/art-20045082

https://www.livescience.com/45090-pregnancy-diet.html